better together*

*This book is best read together, grownup and kid.

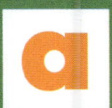 **akidsco.com**

a kids book about

healthy habits

by Trish Turo

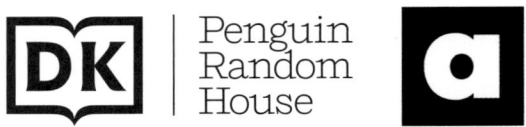

A Kids Co.
Editor Emma Wolf
Designer Rick DeLucco
Creative Director Rick DeLucco
Studio Manager Kenya Feldes
Sales Director Melanie Wilkins
Head of Books Jennifer Goldstein
CEO and Founder Jelani Memory

DK
Senior Production Editor Jennifer Murray
Senior Production Controller Louise Minihane
Senior Acquisitions Editor Katy Flint
Acquisitions Project Editor Sara Forster
Managing Art Editor Vicky Short
Managing Director, Licensing Mark Searle

First American edition, 2025
Published in the United States by DK Publishing, 1745 Broadway, 20th Floor,
New York, NY 10019

First published in Great Britain in 2025 by
Dorling Kindersley Limited, 20 Vauxhall Bridge Road, London SW1V 2SA
A Penguin Random House Company

The authorised representative in the EEA is
Dorling Kindersley Verlag GmbH. Arnulfstr. 124, 80636 Munich, Germany

A catalog record for this book is available from the Library of Congress.
A CIP catalogue record for this book is available from the British Library.
ISBN: 978-0-2417-4309-6

DK books are available at special discounts when purchased in bulk for sales
promotions, premiums, fund-raising, or education use. For details, contact:
DK Publishing Special Markets, 1745 Broadway, 20th Floor, New York, NY 10019
SpecialSales@dk.com

Printed and bound in China
www.dk.com
akidsco.com

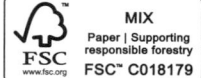

MIX
Paper | Supporting
responsible forestry
FSC™ C018179

This book was made with Forest
Stewardship Council™ certified
paper – one small step in DK's
commitment to a sustainable future.
Learn more at **www.dk.com/uk/
information/sustainability**

To my incredible kids, Dean and Kurt,
who have filled my life with so much gratitude,
growth, and joy. Thank you for continuously
inspiring me, for showing me how to be brave and
most importantly, sharing what unconditional love
looks like. You remind me of what's most important,
and I'll never forget the lessons (and healthy habits!)
you've taught me, and still teach me today.
I love you more than all the galaxies combined!
Love, Mom

Intro
for grownups

Did you know that it only takes one, small step to be well on your way toward your healthiest, happiest life? Did you know habit change is within reach...for you AND your kids? And here's the good news: you don't have to change everything all at once!

One of the best parts of my job is helping people feel empowered to make healthy choices that serve them in their everyday lives. I want to create a world where healthy habits are part of a daily conversation at any age, at any stage. I hope these choices can start to feel simple and effective, and easy to apply in your own life.

In this book, I'll help you and your kids discover the fun of creating healthy habits with a few simple steps, some **SMART** strategies, and some motivation to get started right now.

Let's build some healthy habits together!

Hey, you!

I have some really important
questions to ask you.

Do you ever wonder how you can be your best self **?**

How you can live a happy life **?**

Living your **best, BIGGEST,**

MOST EXCITING LIFE

all comes down to small, **healthy habits**.

Healthy habits are..

....**simple actions you can do every day to celebrate the life you want to live.**

Healthy habits include things like:

getting outside,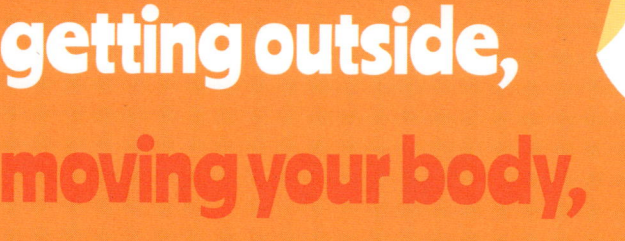
moving your body,
eating yummy foods that fuel you,
getting good sleep,
taking deep breaths,
drinking water,
brushing your teeth,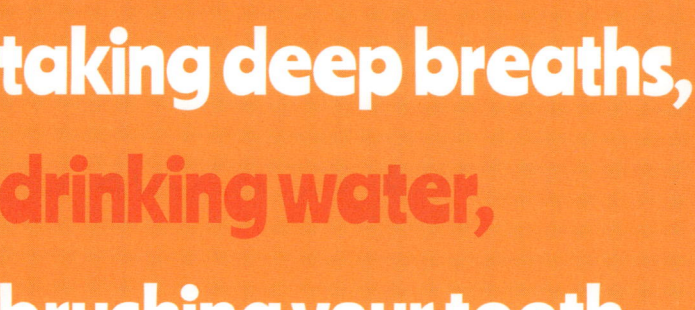
giving warm hugs,
saying kind things to yourself and others...

and the list goes on!

As a health coach, I help people pick which habits to focus on.

A part of the process is talking about what sparks

JOY

and then setting up a plan.

There are a **LOT** of healthy habits to choose from!

Sometimes we can get stuck when trying to narrow our focus to

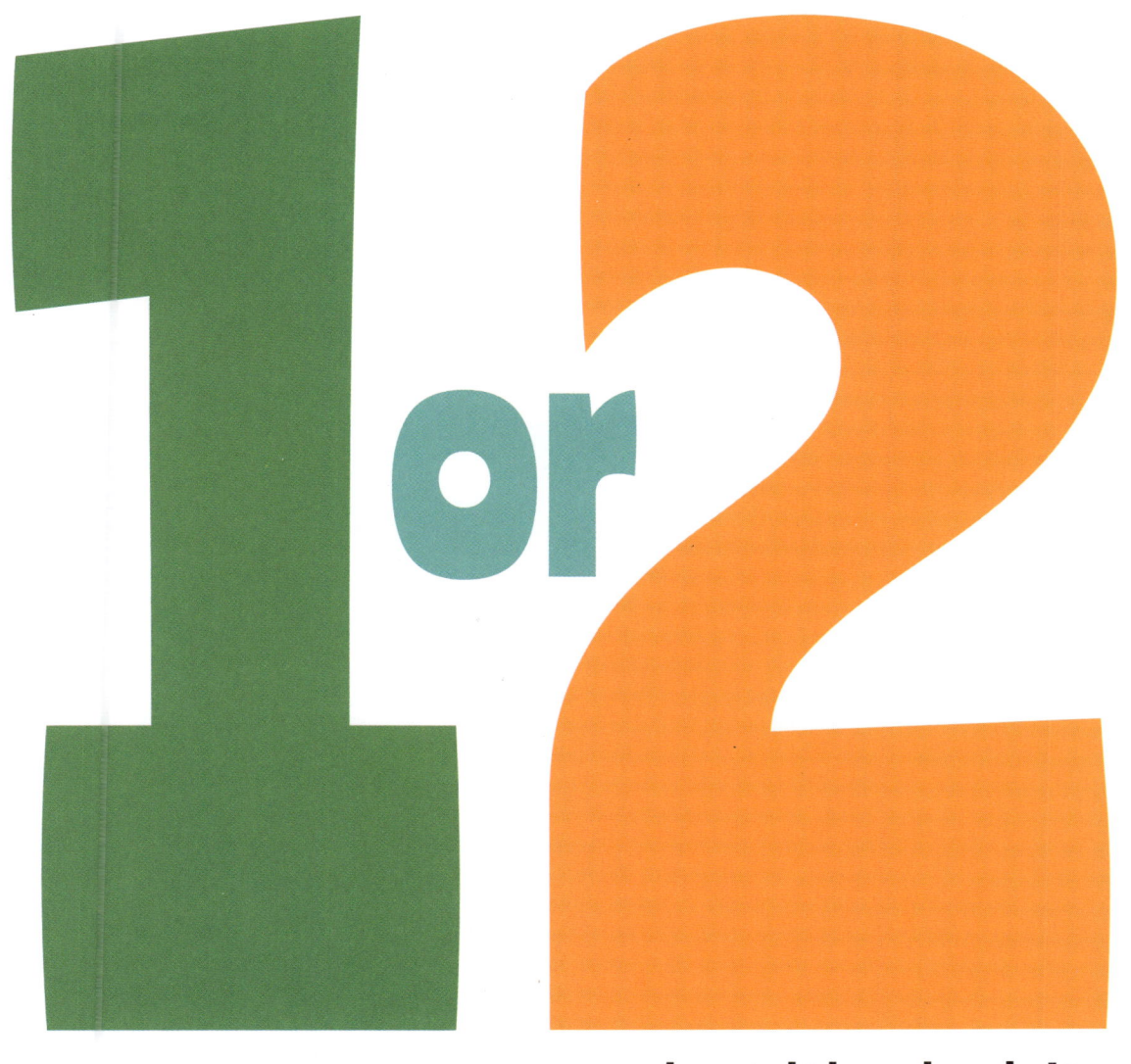

1 or 2

healthy habits.

It's easy to get excited about doing all the things that make our brains light up and say,

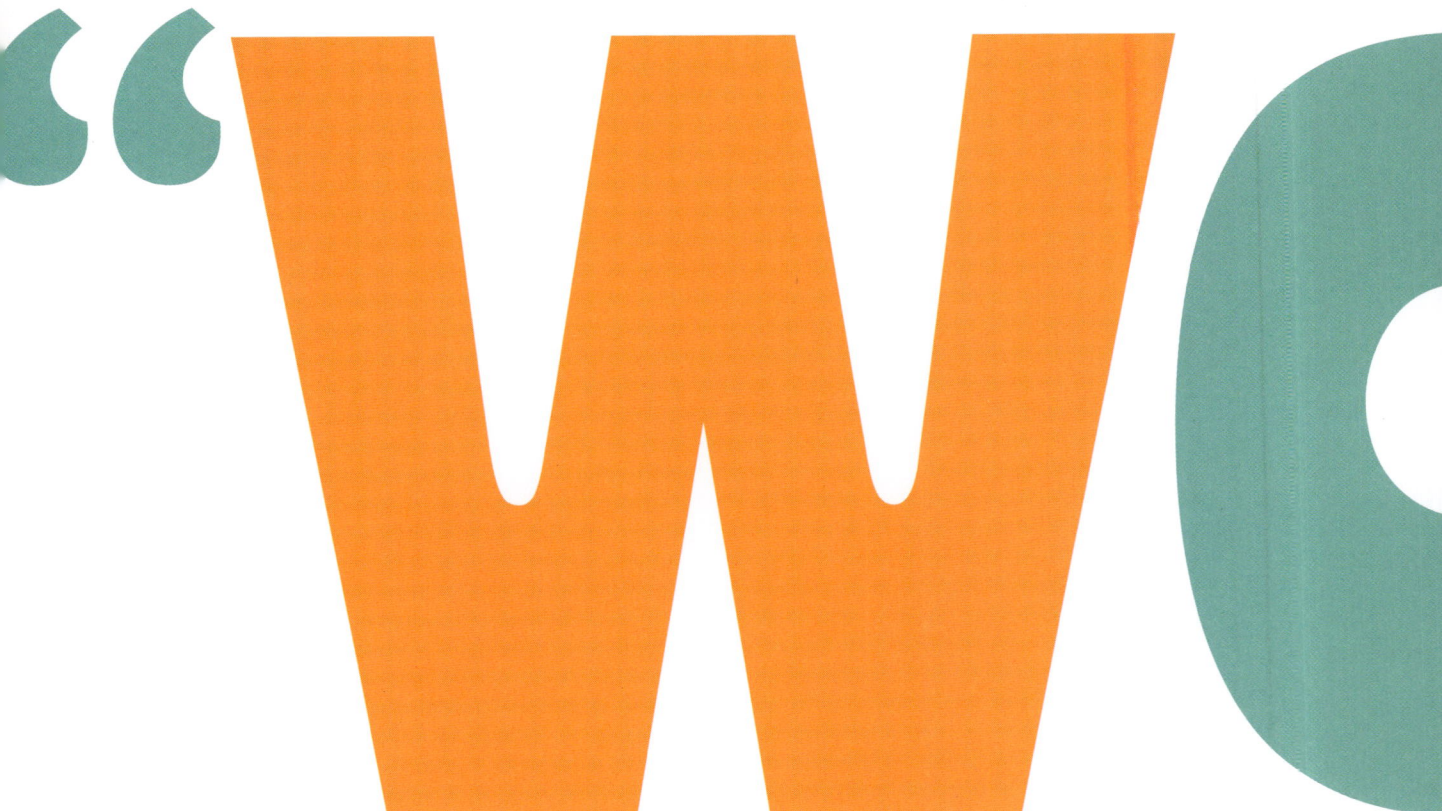

"W

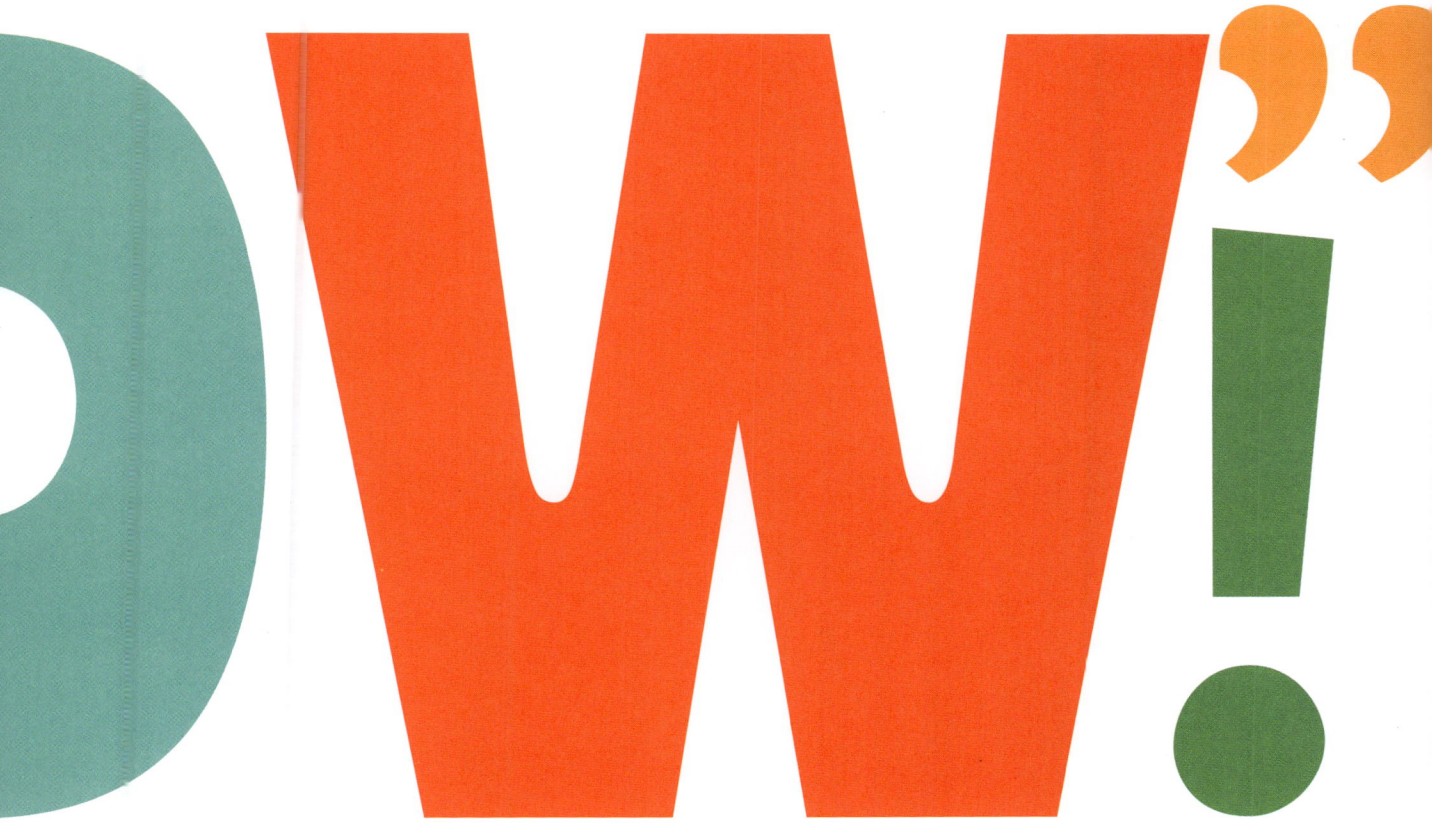

But when the list is too long, we may get frustrated or overwhelmed...and then we might not do anything at all!

While our brains are great at helping us solve problems, doing a LOT all at the SAME TIME can make us feel stuck.

And when we feel stuck, we might even start practicing habits that *aren't* helpful.

This can look like:

spending too much time inside,
moving our bodies less,
eating foods that don't help our bodies,
not getting enough sleep or sleeping too much,
forgetting to breathe,
not drinking enough water,
not brushing our teeth,
staying away from others for a long time,
saying unkind things to ourselves and others...

and unfortunately, this list can go on as well.

So, what
do we do?

If you feel unsure, excited, overwhelmed—or all of these things at once—you aren't alone, and I have some ideas for you!

The truth is, being your healthiest self is easiest when you make small, simple, joy-filled choices, every day.

There's a helpful term to think about when making healthy habits:

a SMART goal.

Our **SMART** brains love helpful reminders to keep us on track...

and **SMART** goals are behaviors put into action that set us up for success.

Let's get into it!

The S in SMART stands for specific.

This means the habit you're building should be clear.

This looks like,

"I will walk around the block,"

instead of,

"I will move more."

It's descriptive!

The M in SMART stands for measurable.

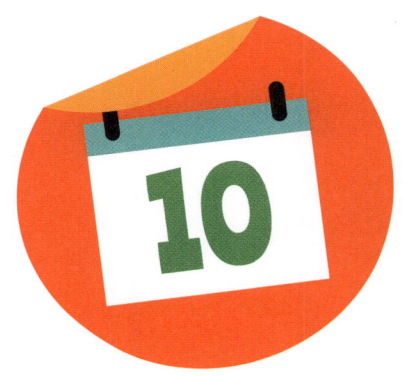

This means the habit you're building has a set value.

This could be a number of days per week, or a certain amount of minutes per day.

The A in SMART stands for achievable.

This means your healthy habit sets you up for success!

Is your goal one you can feel accomplished in doing?

The R in SMART stands for realistic.

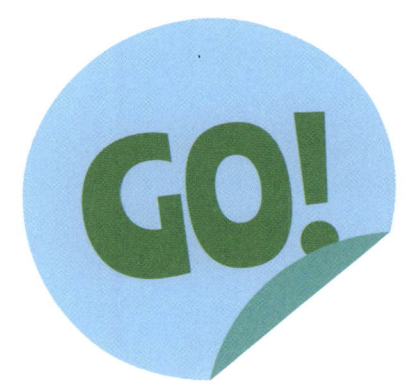

This means your healthy habit is something you can start right now.

In this moment, what is something you can do for your well-being?

The T in SMART stands for timely.

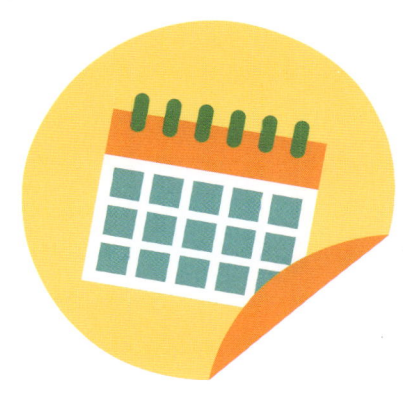

And this means your healthy habit is something you can accomplish within a set time frame.

Maybe you try something for a day, a week, or even a whole month.

You get to decide!

Making **SMART** goals is a tool I use with people who are ready to make changes, and need support.

Now, it's a tool you can use, too!

I invite you to pick 1 healthy habit you want to try.

Think of 1 or 2 small things that sound interesting to you. Then ask yourself...

What motivates me?
Why do I want to do this?
Why is this important to me?

A healthy habit can sound like this:

"To help my brain grow, I will spend 10 minutes outside, every day."

Or, like this:

"To help me grow strong, I will do an activity that moves my body every day."

Or even like this:

"To help me feel ready to sleep, I will brush my teeth and get in bed at the same time every night."

Is this starting to make sense? **Yay!**

Now, I encourage you to get a sticky note or piece of paper and write down your goal when you have it.

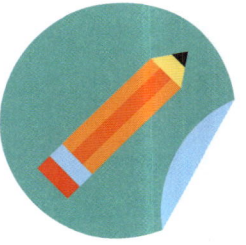

Then, put that goal somewhere you can see it every day!

By your bed, taped to your bathroom mirror, in your daily planner or journal. Maybe you even write it on the back of your hand!

I want you to be successful
in creating your best, biggest,
most exciting life.

So, let's get all the help we can get!

Tell a grownup. Tell a friend.
Tell someone special to you.

Share your **SMART** goal with someone else, and ask them what goals they're working on!

Then, you can support and motivate each other as you work toward your goals.

OK!

Now, you've learned the importance and power of simple, healthy choices.

I can't wait for you

to live your best life!

What healthy are you

habits.

excited to create?

Outro
for grownups

Congratulations! You're already well on your way to becoming a healthy habit expert! Here are some ways to keep healthy habits a part of your daily conversations:

*Ask yourself **why** it's important to you.*

Understanding your "why" is helpful to evaluate whether you're ready to take meaningful steps toward habit-building. Your "why" should spark joy and light you up!

Start small and simple.

Our brains can only do so much when it comes to creating an action plan. It's critical to start small and stick with it so that your choices turn into a real habit versus a one-off thing.

Make it fun.

The things that are fun, engaging, and interesting are ones we'll want to do over and over. Every habit isn't necessarily fun right away. But add an accountability buddy and rewards to look forward to, and the process feels more enjoyable!

Consistency is key—use that **SMART** brain of yours to come up with some healthy habits and get started today!

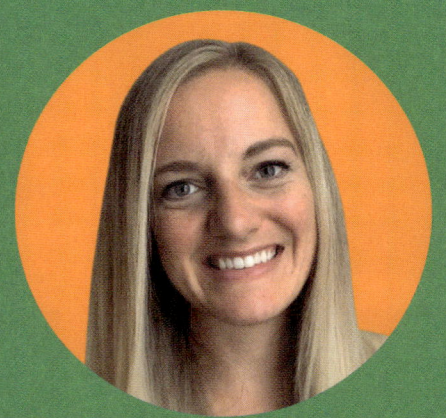

About The Author

Trish Turo (she/her) is a brain health researcher, coach, and healthy habit expert. She has her master's in health psychology and is a national board-certified health and wellness coach. She supports people in all kinds of healthy habits from moving, eating, and sleeping well, to reducing stress and using brain health tools to support cognitive function. Trish has worked with kids and grownups across the lifespan to help people understand that you can build a happy, healthy life at any age, and any stage.

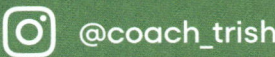 @coach_trish   @trish-turo-health